D1062056

# 30-Minute Yoga

Copyright © 2011 by Viveka Blom Nygren
Photographs copyright © 2011 by David Loftus
First published by Nygren & Nygren as *30 Minuters Yoga*, Sweden 2009
Published by agreement with Norstedts Agency
Translation by Blake Jason Boulerice

Skyhorse Publishing books may be purchased in bulk at special discounts for sales promotion, corporate gifts, fund-raising, or educational purposes. Special editions can also be created to specifications. For details, contact the Special Sales Department, Skyhorse Publishing, 307 West 36th Street, 11th Floor, New York, NY 10018 or info@skyhorsepublishing.com.

www.skyhorsepublishing.com

10 9 8 7 6 5 4 3 2 1

Library of Congress Cataloging-in-Publication Data

Nygren, Viveka Blom.
  30-minute yoga: for better balance and strength in your life / Viveka Blom Nygren.
      p. cm.
  Thirty minute yoga
  ISBN 978-1-61608-064-8 (hardcover: alk. paper)
  1. Astanga yoga. I. Title. II. Title: Thirty minute yoga.
   RA781.68.N94 2011
   613.7'046—dc22
                                        2010033651

Printed in China

30-Minute

# Yoga

### For Better Balance
### and Strength in
### Your Life

Viveka Blom Nygren          Photographs by David Loftus

Skyhorse Publishing

# Contents

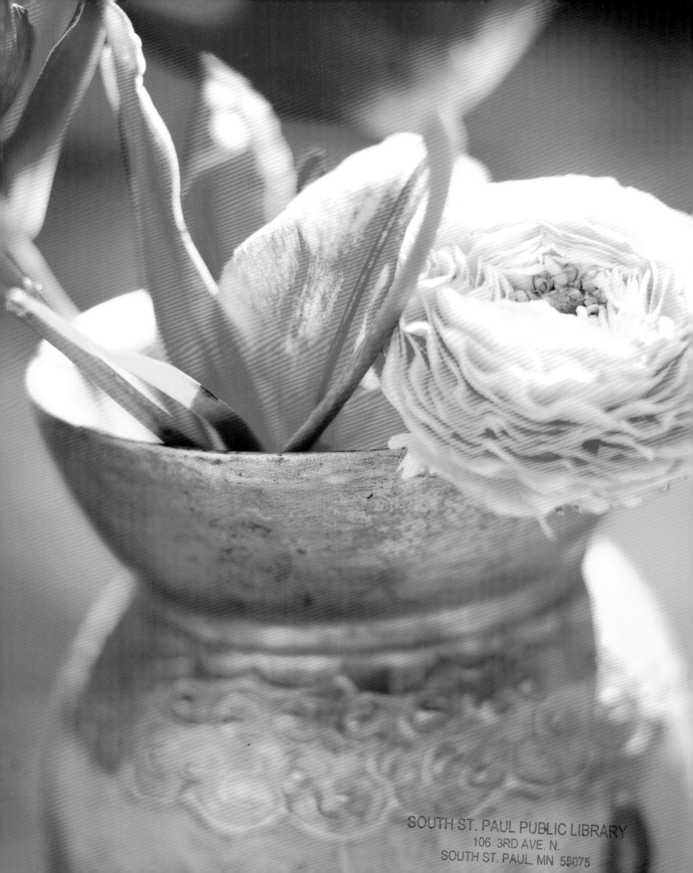

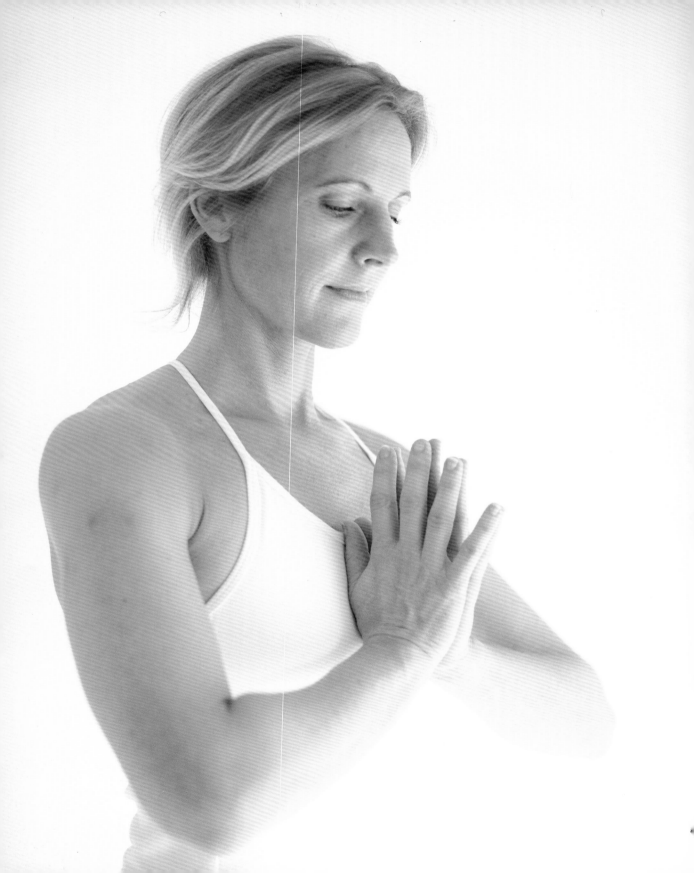

# Foreword

YOGA IS A LIFE PHILOSOPHY that teaches you to find your inner wisdom. It helps you to live your life in harmony with both yourself and the world around you. For many thousands of years, people have practiced yoga in the form of movements, breathing, and meditation to keep the body healthy, to relax the mind, and to achieve focus in life. Often we live entirely in our heads, the mind is overloaded, and the body is left behind. In yoga you use your body as a tool to reach into yourself and to find the power we all carry inside us. Through breathing and moving your body, you can acquire balance among your heart, brain, body, and soul. The body becomes flexible and strong, and your mind becomes more focused and calm, making you happier and more content with yourself.

Here you will receive instructions on how to perform a shorter yoga session in 30 minutes at home when you do not have the time or the opportunity to go to a yoga studio. The book can be used by both beginners and more experienced practitioners. For the beginner, modifications (easier variants) of the complete movement are shown, making this a starting point in your practice of yoga. For the veteran practitioner, this makes for a shorter yoga session that can be done at home on days when you are not doing your full yoga sequence. The yoga positions are taken from the most dynamic form of yoga, Ashtanga Vinyasa Yoga, and are freely arranged for a shorter yoga session.

Om Shanti

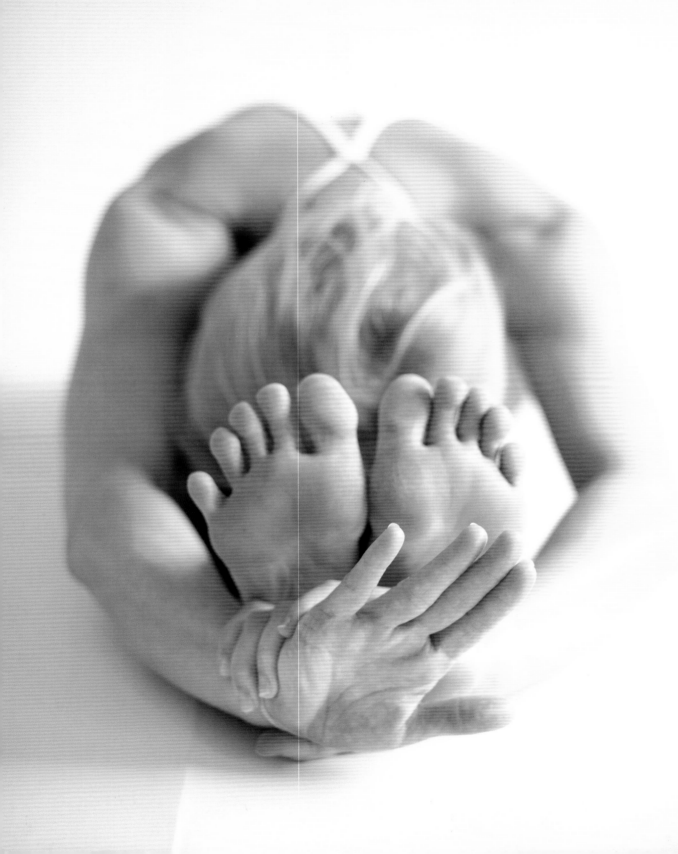

# Practicing yoga

FOR THOSE WHO HAVE NOT PRACTICED yoga before, my first recommendation is to try to find a routine that fits in with your daily life. It is better to do a little yoga often than a lot only now and then. You may begin by doing the sun salutations and working with them for some weeks, each or every other morning, or at some other time of day that suits you. After that you can build on the sequence and add movements to it. When all the movements have been performed, this yoga session will take you approximately 30 minutes to complete. Each movement is described in both text and in pictures, with and without modifications. The pictures help you to get it right and to build up to the full movement. Use the modification until you feel comfortable going further. If you do yoga often, three or more times per week, you will be able to drop the modification after approximately two to three months.

FOR THOSE WHO ARE VETERAN yoga practitioners, this book can be used as a shorter session that you can perform at home daily. My advice to you is to try to make yoga a part of your life, from which you can gather focus, strength, and calm. On those days when you cannot set aside 30 minutes, you can either sit and breathe to yourself for a while or do the sun salutations.

I hope that this book will be able to inspire you to do the movements with greater precision, and that you will find support from the various modifications that are provided.

IT IS ADVISED to do yoga first thing in the morning, on an empty stomach, and with an empty mind. However, it is better to do yoga at some other time of day than not at all. Try to avoid eating approximately two hours before you do yoga. Always listen to your body, and do nothing that feels forced or that causes pain. Each day is new, and your breathing and movements will feel different depending on how you have eaten and slept, and on where you are in your hormonal cycle. Women should avoid doing yoga during the first three days of menstruation as well as avoid upward-and-downward movements. Pregnant women should perform specially adapted pregnant yoga.

FIND A WARM and quiet place in which to do yoga. You need a yoga mat so as not to slip on the floor or carpet. Use soft, preferably light-fitting clothing that is easy to move around in. In this book, the names of the movements are given in Sanskrit, which is an ancient Indic language, but the words are also found translated into English.

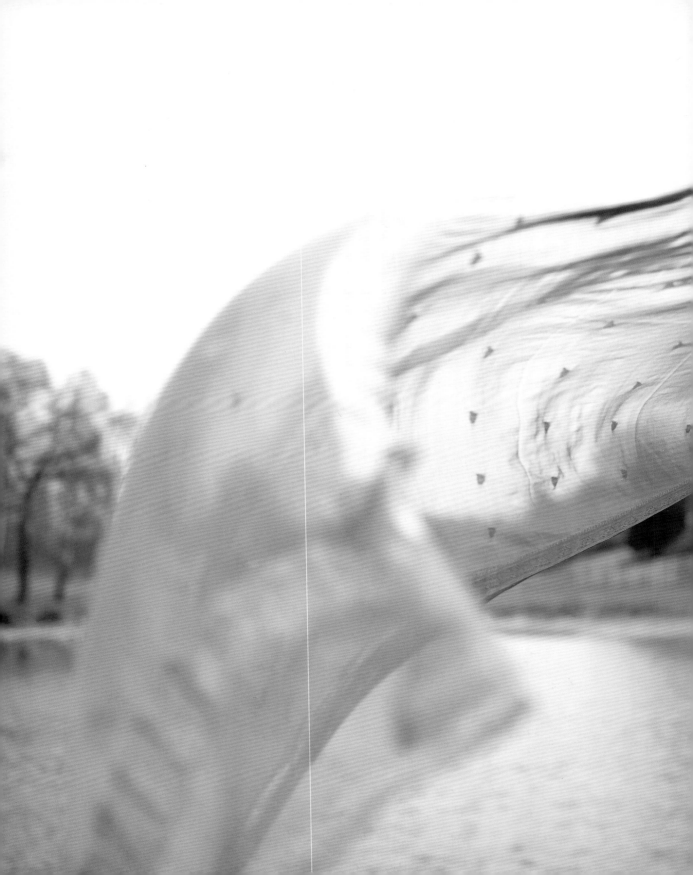

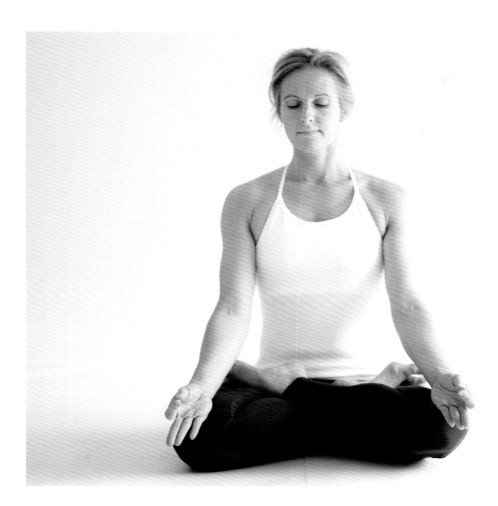

# Breathing

– UJJAY PRANAYAMA

To breathe is to live. Normally we use only a small part of our lung capacity when we breathe. In yoga you will learn to breathe deeply. When you breathe deeply and calmly, you warm the body, get the energy flowing, and relax the mind. Breathing is the foundation of yoga, and it is born out of movement.

1. Sit down on the yoga mat with legs crossed. To begin you may need a blanket or pillow under your bottom. 2. Stretch your back upward and keep your shoulders lowered in line with your hips. Your spine should be as straight as possible in order to give your lungs greater breathing space. 3. Close your mouth and breathe through your nose, and collect your breath at the back of the throat. A gentle hissing sound can be heard, as in deep sleep. 4. Breathe in and fill your lungs completely so that your thorax expands. 5. When you breathe out again, you feel your chest sink slowly back. Try to empty your lungs completely when exhaling, thereby prolonging and deepening your breath. Listen to your breathing for a while, and let go of any thoughts that surround you. Follow a journey of discovery in your body, and let breathing be your mantra during the yoga session. Feel how breathing gives life and energy to every cell in your body.

# The body lock

In yoga you work with both small and large muscles in the body. What may feel new and unfamiliar is that you must have contact with your inner, deeper abdominal muscles. In yoga this is called "root lock"—*mula bandha*—and "abdominal lock"—*uddiyana bandha*. These body locks steer the flow of energy in your body, and they also give the body good support when you move in harmony with your breathing. These locks must create an inner, rising energy that is your power and the center of your body. When you engage the root lock, you raise the perineum and all the small muscles at the base of the pelvis, and you keep the buttocks relaxed and feel an inner lift. It is a small movement. You then draw the deep abdominal muscles just below the navel inward and back toward your spine, almost as though to embrace your lower back. When these locks are engaged, the diaphragm is lifted up into the body so that your abdomen is completely still when you breathe. Instead it is your stomach and chest that accompany your breathing. When you engage your feet, by spreading your toes and feeling a lift in the arch, you automatically gain contact with your leg muscles, which also puts you in contact with the root and abdominal locks. If in the beginning it feels difficult to find the root and abdominal locks, it will suffice to concentrate on having stronger feet and stronger legs. What is important is that you feel a connection with the center of your body.

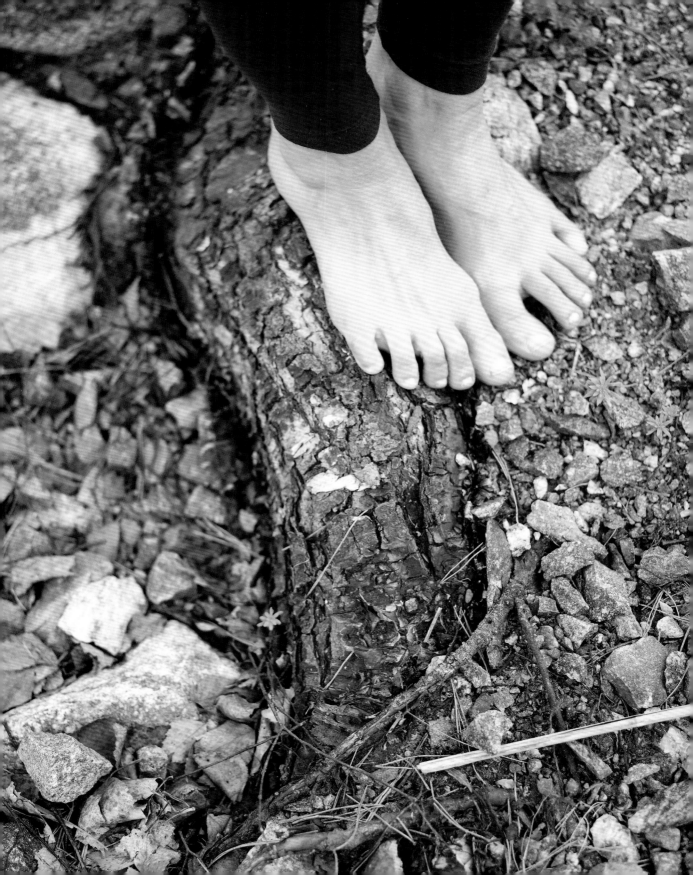

# Yoga movements
## –ASANAS

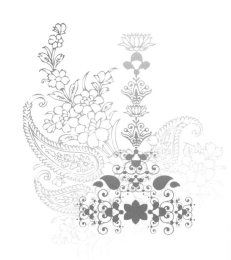

# Mountain pose

– SAMASTITIHI
You must try to imitate this position in all the yoga poses you do, regardless of whether you are extending your arms or your legs, or bending forward or backward. Strive to have contact with the center of your body, and to achieve balance between it and your breathing.

1.  Stand with your feet together, let your big toes touch one another, and leave possibly a few inches between the heels. Here your body is in balance. Feel contact with your toes, feet, legs, and deep abdominals.

2.  Raise your chest, lower your shoulders, and gently draw your tailbone in below you so that your lower back is level. The back of your neck is in line with your spine, and you rise up with the top of your head toward the sky.

3.  Breathing that is deep and calm warms and gets the energy flowing throughout your entire body.

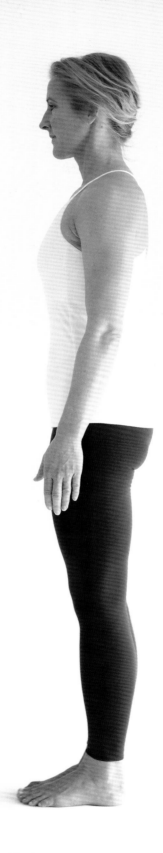

# Sun salutation A

– SURYANAMASKARA

This pose cleanses the mind, and warms and strengthens the body. This is a tribute to the sun, which is the greatest creative power in nature—that which gives us energy.

The Sun salutations are done in a sequence in which each part of the movement has an in- or exhalation. Take extra breaths where you need to. In the *Dog* position, which is the main position in the Sun salutations, you stand for five breaths. The Sun salutations are powerful, and it takes a while for the body to get used to them. Whenever you feel the need to, rest in the *Child's pose*, which is described on page 57.

1. Stand in the *Mountain pose*.

2. Breathe in, and stretch your arms forward and up over your head. Keep the palms of your hands together, and look toward your thumbs.

3. Breathe out, let your upper body fall forward, and place your palms on the floor directly in front of your feet. If you need to, keep your knees slightly bent. Draw your shoulder blades into your body so that your shoulders are far from your ears, with your head facing down toward the floor.

4. Breathe in, open your chest, and stretch your head upward, keeping your hands on the floor.

5. Breathe out, and step or jump a leg's length back. Push your upper body forward, and keep your elbows beside your body while lowering your body toward the floor. If this is too difficult, place your knees on the floor. Try to stop before your entire body is on the floor. It is important that you are strong in your legs and that you hold your position so that you do not lose contact with the center of your body. Do not raise your buttocks or arch your back. This position is called the *Plank*.

*Continued on the next page.*

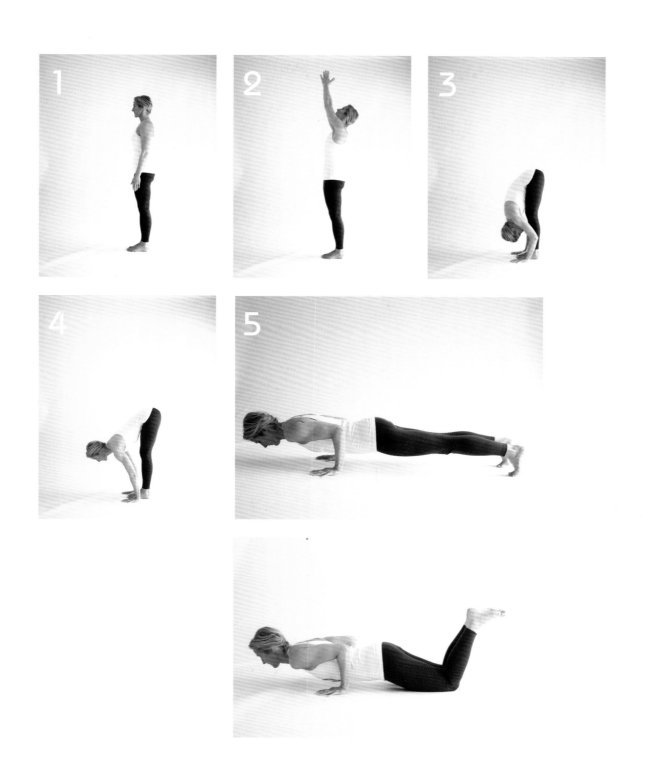

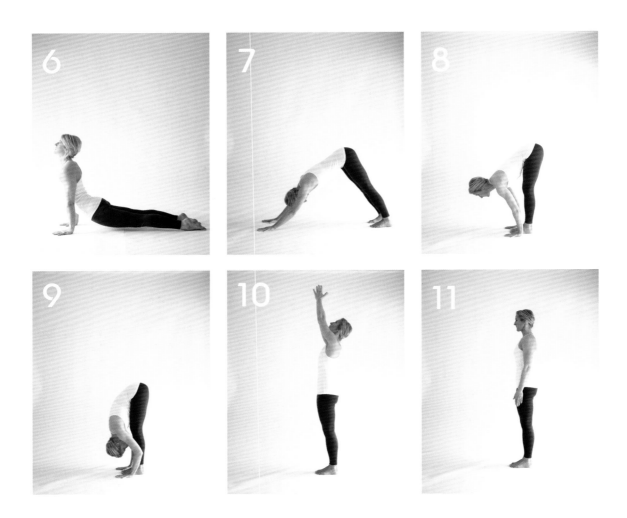

6.  Breathe in, and roll over on your toes so that the top of the foot lies against the floor. Press down with your hands and arms so that you rise up with arms straight. Stretch your upper body upward, and open your chest by pressing your sternum forward. Keep your shoulders lowered, and draw your shoulder blades deep into your body. Keep the width of your hips between your feet, and be strong in your legs. This position is called the *Upward-facing dog*.

7.  Breathe out, roll over on your toes, and raise your hips. Place your feet on the floor with your hips up and back and your head facing downward. Try to keep your hands and feet in the same place as they were in the *Upward-facing dog*. Keep your hands shoulder-width apart, and spread your fingers. Your index finger should point straight ahead, and your entire palm should be on the floor. Keep your feet hips-width apart and, if you need to, bend your knees slightly. Keep the back of your neck in line with your spine, and let your head hang freely. Broaden your shoulders, press against the floor with strong arms, and hold this position for five deep breaths. This position is called the *Dog* or the *Downward-facing dog*.

8.  Breathe in, and jump or step forward, keeping the palms of your hands on the floor. Open your chest, and stretch your head upward, keeping your knees bent if you need to. Keep your feet together.

9.  Breathe out, let your head fall downward, and keep your hands on the floor.

10. Breathe in, and be strong in your legs. Leading with your chest, rise all the way up with arms over your head and palms together, and look toward your thumbs.

11. Breathe out, and come down with your arms alongside your body and back to the *Mountain pose*.

12. Repeat this sequence three times.

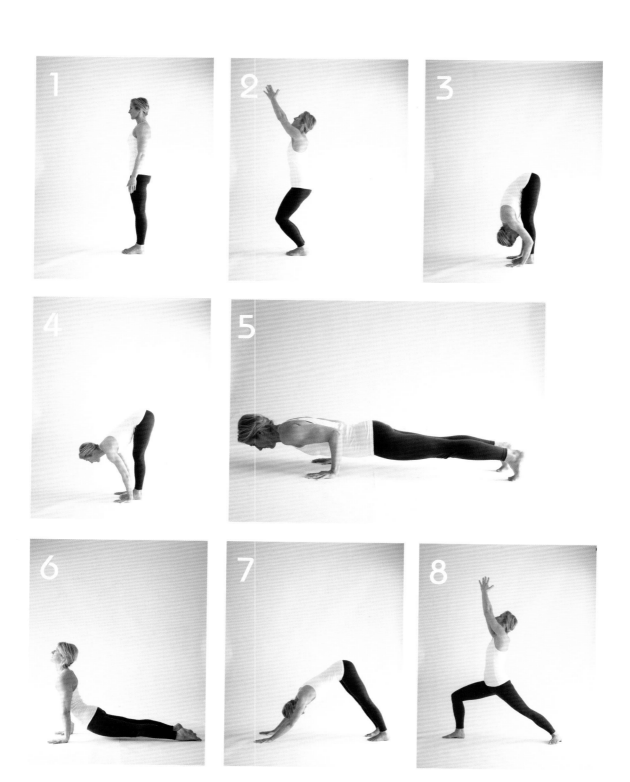

# Sun salutation ß

1.  Stand in the *Mountain pose*.

2.  Breathe in, bend your knees deeply, and stretch your arms forward and up over your head. Keep the palms of your hands together, and look toward your thumbs.

3.  Breathe out, let your upper body fall forward, and place your palms on the floor directly in front of your feet. If you need to, keep your knees slightly bent. Draw your shoulder blades into your body so that your shoulders are far from your ears, with your head facing down toward the floor.

4.  Breathe in, open your chest, and stretch your head upward, keeping your hands on the floor.

5.  Breathe out, step or jump a leg's length back, and come down to the *Plank*.

6.  Breathe in, roll over on your toes, and rise up to the *Upward-facing dog*.

7.  Breathe out, raise your hips, place your feet on the floor, and rise up to the *Downward-facing dog* with your hips up and back and your head facing downward.

8.  Breathe in, and turn your left heel so that your foot is approximately at a 45-degree angle to an imaginary line along the middle of the mat. Lift your right foot forward, and place it behind your right thumb. If your foot gets caught, grip your leg and lift below your knee to get your leg forward. Keep your knee at a 90-degree angle. Raise your arms up over your head with palms together, and look toward your thumbs. Be strong in your back leg.

*Continued on the next page.*

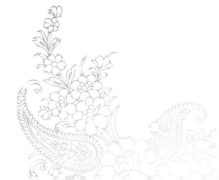

9. Breathe out, and lift your right leg back. Push your upper body forward, and keep your elbows beside your body while lowering your body toward the floor. If this is too difficult, place your knees on the floor.

10. Breathe in, and press down with your hands and arms so that you rise to the *Upward-facing dog*.

11. Breathe out, raise your hips, place your feet on the floor, and rise up to the *Downward-facing dog* with your hips up and back and your head facing downward.

12. Breathe in, and turn your right heel so that your foot is approximately at a 45-degree angle to an imaginary line along the middle of the mat. Lift your left foot forward, and place it behind your left thumb. If your foot gets caught, grip your leg and lift below your knee to get your leg forward. Keep your knee at a 90-degree angle. Raise your arms up over your head with palms together, and look toward your thumbs. Be strong in your back leg.

13. Breathe out, lift your left leg back, and push your upper body forward. Keep your elbows beside your body while lowering your body toward the floor, and place your knees on the floor if you need to.

14. Breathe in, and press down with your hands and arms so that you rise up to the *Upward-facing dog*.

15. Breathe out, roll over on your toes, and raise your hips. Place your feet on the floor, and rise up to the *Downward-facing dog* with your hips up and back and your head facing downward. Try to keep your hands and feet in the same place as they were in the *Upward-facing dog*. Keep your hands shoulder-width apart, and spread your fingers. Your index finger should point straight ahead, and your entire palm should be on the floor. Keep your feet hips-width apart, and, if you need to, bend your knees slightly. Keep the back of your neck in line with your spine, and let your head hang freely. Broaden your shoulders, press against the floor with strong arms, and hold this position for five deep breaths.

16. Breathe in, and jump or step forward, keeping the palms of your hands on the floor. Open your chest, and stretch your head upward, keeping your knees bent if you need to. Keep your feet together.

17. Breathe out, let your head fall downward, and keep your hands on the floor.

18. Breathe in, bend your knees deeply, and rise all the way up with arms over your head and palms together, looking toward your thumbs and keeping your knees bent.

19. Breathe out, and return to the *Mountain pose* with legs straight and arms by your sides.

20. Repeat this sequence three times.

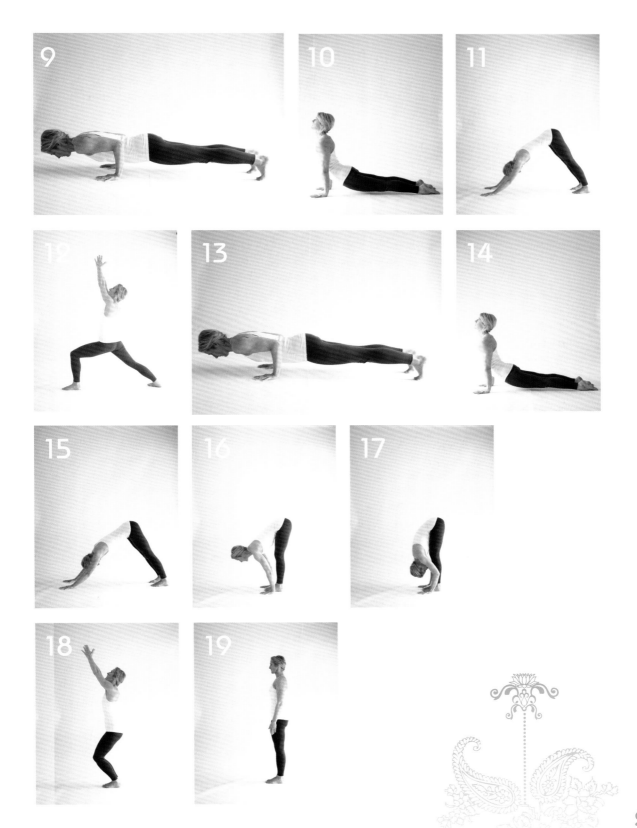

The following are several movements in which you step out to the right. Each movement begins and ends in the Mountain pose.

# Triangle pose and reverse triangle pose

– UTTHITA TRIKONASANA AND PARIVRITTA TRIKONASANA
Strengthens and stretches the legs, back, and feet, and opens the hips and chest. Prevents and relieves back and neck pain.

1. Stand in the *Mountain pose*.

2. Breathe in, and step a leg's length to the right. Extend your arms with palms facing downward. Your heels should be in line, and make sure that your toes point straight ahead. Be strong in your feet and legs. Avoid locking your knee by keeping it slightly bent, thereby working your leg muscles without weighing on your knees or joints. Turn your right foot out at a 90-degree angle. Make sure that your toes point straight out, and keep your knees and thighs in line. Lift your left heel back a bit.

3. Breathe out, and extend your right side over your right leg. Lower your hand and grasp your ankle, and gradually reach for your big toe. Look down toward your right foot and make sure that your shoulders and upper body are in line with your right leg. Raise your left arm up toward the ceiling, and look up toward your left hand. Do not lean forward or backward, and try to keep the line with your right leg all the way up to your left arm. Hold this position for five deep breaths.

4. Breathe in, and rise up on parallel feet with arms extended.

5. Breathe out, turn your left foot out at a 90-degree angle, and now repeat the movement on your left side.

6. Breathe in, and rise up on parallel feet with arms extended.

7. Breathe out, turn your right foot out again at a 90-degree angle, lift your left heel back a bit, and push your left hip forward so that your hips are as parallel as possible. Come down with your left hand at shoulder-width beside your right foot. Then gradually place your hand outside your right foot. Rise up with your

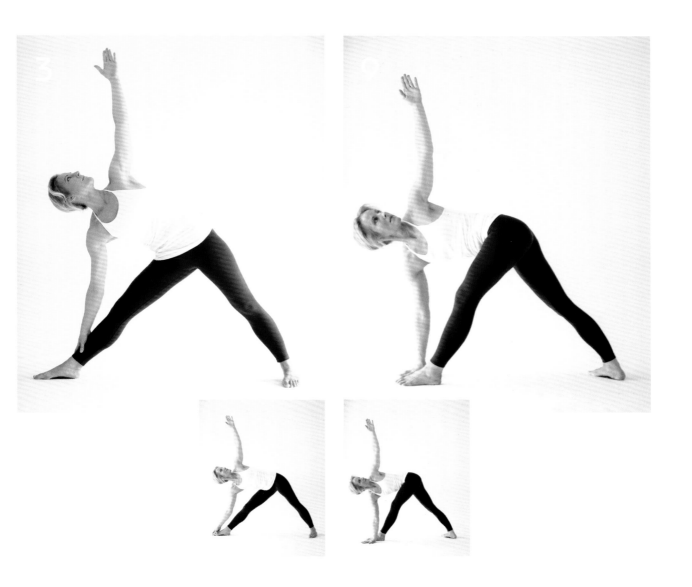

right hand toward the ceiling, turn fully at the waist, and look up toward your right hand. Hold this position for five deep breaths.

8.  Breathe in, rise up on parallel feet, and extend your arms.

9.  Breathe out, turn your left foot out at a 90-degree angle, and now repeat the movement on your left side.

10. Breathe in, and rise up on parallel feet with arms extended.

11. Breathe in, and return to the *Mountain pose*.

# Extended side angle pose

– UTTHITA PARSCHVAKONASANA

Strengthens the back, hips, ankles, and legs, and opens the hips and chest. Counteracts sciatica and facilitates digestion.

1. Stand in the *Mountain pose*.

2. Breathe in, step wide out to the right, and extend your arms. Your heels should be in line, and your toes should point straight ahead. Have strong feet and legs.

3. Breathe out, and turn your right foot out at a 90-degree angle. Make sure that your toes point straight out, and keep your knees and thighs in line. Bend your right knee over your right foot at a 90-degree angle. Place your right arm on your right knee, and then gradually place your right hand down outside your right foot. Open the side of your body toward the ceiling. Take your left arm out from under, and stretch your arm forward and over your body. Try to stabilize your shoulders by drawing the shoulder blades deep into the body. Look up under your left arm, and keep the back of your neck in line with your spine. Keep your back leg steady on the floor with your back foot strong so that you do not weigh down on your right knee. Maintain balance between your front and back feet. Hold this position for five deep breaths.

4. Breathe in, and rise up on parallel feet with arms extended. Turn your left foot out at a 90-degree angle, and repeat the movement on your left side.

5. Breathe in, and rise up on parallel feet with arms extended.

6. Breathe out, and return to the *Mountain pose*.

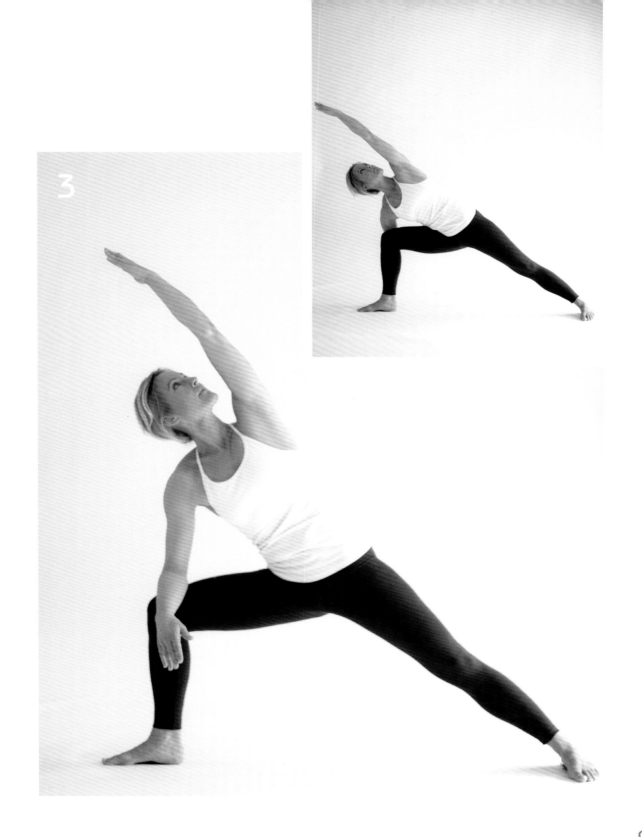

3

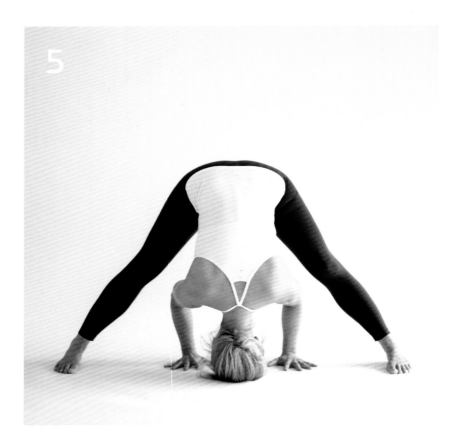

5

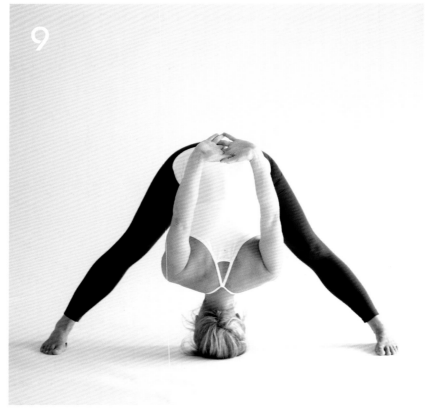

9

# Wide-legged forward bend

– PRASARITA PADOTTANASANA

Stretches and strengthens the back of your legs. Increases circulation to the head and trunk which, among other things, promotes digestion.

1. Stand in the *Mountain pose*.

2. Breathe in, and jump or step a leg's length to the right. Place your hands on your waist. Your heels should be in line, and make sure that your toes point straight ahead. Be strong in your feet and legs. Avoid locking your knees by keeping them minimally bent, thereby working your leg muscles without weighing on your knees or hips. Open your chest.

3. Breathe out, let your upper body fall forward, and place your hands on the floor shoulder-width apart. Bend your knees slightly if you need to.

4. Breathe in, straighten your arms, and stretch your head upward.

5. Breathe out, and let your upper body fall forward with your head facing down toward the floor. Be strong in your feet and legs, stretch out your back, and hold this position for five deep breaths.

6. Breathe in, straighten your arms, and stretch your head upward. Keep steady, and breathe out.

7. Breathe in, come all the way up, and breathe out.

8. Breathe in, and extend your arms. Move your hands behind your back, and fold your hands.

9. Breathe out, let your back fall forward with your head facing downward, and extend your arms as much as you can. Be strong in your legs and feet, and hold this position for five deep breaths.

10. Breathe in, and come all the way up with hands folded behind your back. Breathe out.

11. Breathe in, and return to the *Mountain pose*.

# Warrior pose 1 and 2

– VIRABHADRASANA

Strengthens your ankles, knees, legs, hips, back, and lower abdomen. Supports the organs in the core and gives greater balance in the body.

### WARRIOR POSE 1

1. Stand in the *Mountain pose*.

2. Breathe in, and step wide out to the right with arms extended. Turn your right foot out at a 90-degree angle with your toes pointing straight ahead. Turn your left heel so that your foot is at a 45-degree angle to an imaginary line along the middle of the mat. Push your left hip forward so that your hips are as parallel as possible.

3. Breathe out, and bend your right knee at a 90-degree angle over your right foot. Keep your back leg strong, and try to keep your back foot entirely on the floor. Push your left hip forward, and draw your right hip back, so that you have balance in the movement and do not weigh forward on your right knee. Stretch your arms above your head with palms together. Look toward your thumbs. Hold this position for five breaths.

4. Breathe in, and come back on parallel feet, keeping your arms above your head. Breathe out, turn your left foot out at a 90-degree angle, and now repeat the movement on your left side.

### WARRIOR POSE 2

5. Breathe out, and keep your left knee at a 90-degree angle. Extend your arms at shoulder-height with palms facing downward. Open your hips to the side, and turn your back foot forward a bit. Draw your tailbone in below you so that you do not raise your buttocks. Keep your upper body straight up from the hips to avoid weighing forward. Be strong in both legs so that you have balance in the movement. Take five breaths, and look toward your left hand's fingertips.

6. Breathe in, and come back on parallel feet with arms extended. Breathe out, turn your right foot out at a 90-degree angle, and now repeat the movement on your right side.

7. Breathe in, and come back on parallel feet with arms extended. Breathe out, and return to the *Mountain pose*.

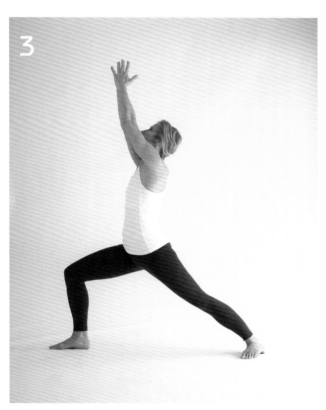

WARRIOR POSE 1

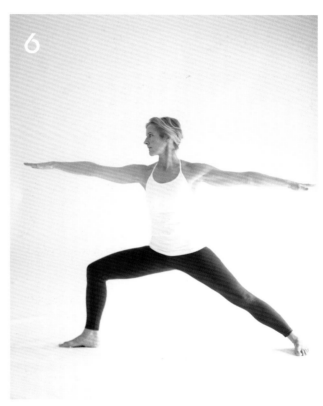

WARRIOR POSE 2

31

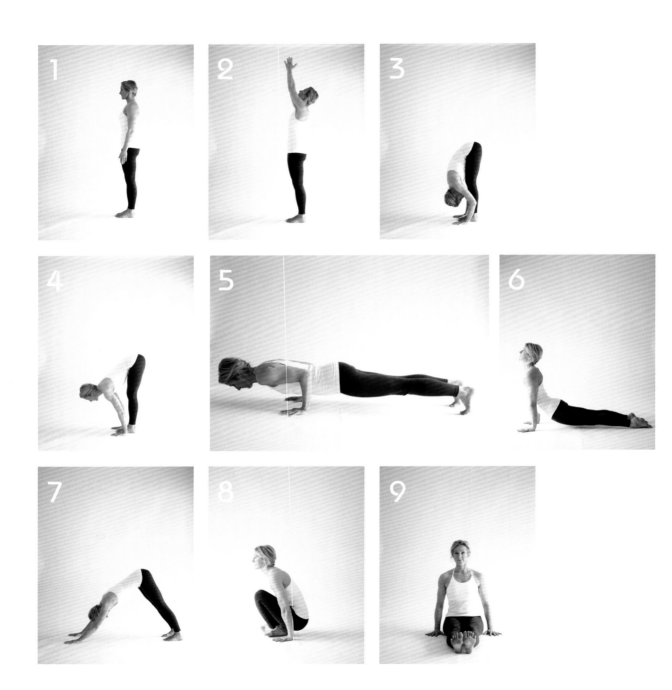

# Vinyasa to seated movements

1. Stand in the *Mountain pose*.

2. Breathe in, and stretch your arms forward and up over your head. Keep the palms of your hands together, and look toward your thumbs.

3. Breathe out, let your upper body fall forward, and place your palms on the floor directly in front of your feet. If you need to, keep your knees slightly bent. Draw your shoulder blades into your body so that your shoulders are far from your ears, with your head facing down toward the floor.

4. Breathe in, open your chest, and stretch your head upward, keeping your hands on the floor.

5. Breathe out, step or jump a leg's length back, and come down to the *Plank*.

6. Breathe in, and rise up to the *Upward-facing dog*.

7. Breathe out, roll over on your toes, and raise your hips. Place your feet on the floor, and rise up to the *Downward-facing dog* with your hips up and back and your head facing downward.

8. Breathe in, bend your knees, and jump or step forward to seated position with legs crossed.

9. Here begins the seated sequence. The starting position is sitting with hips parallel, back straight, active extended legs, and feet together.

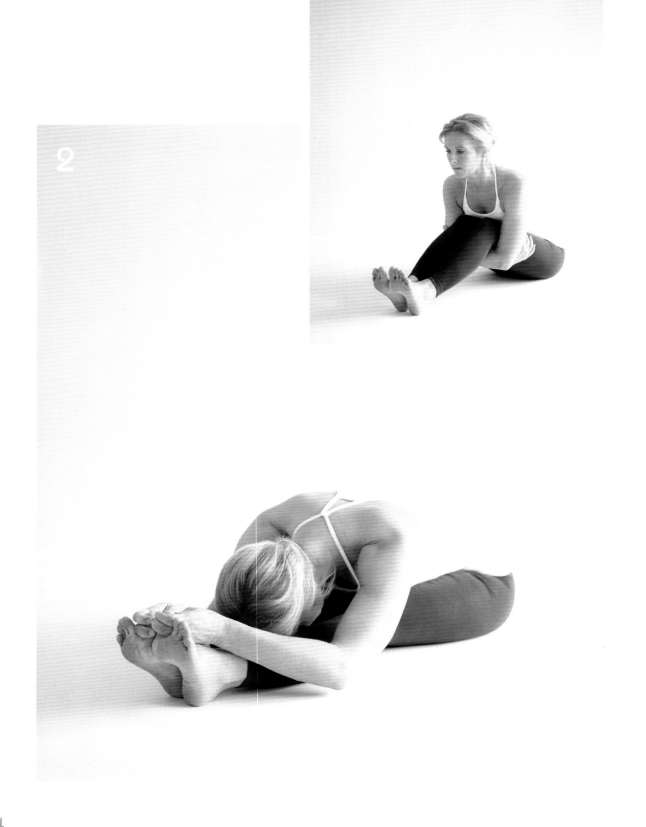

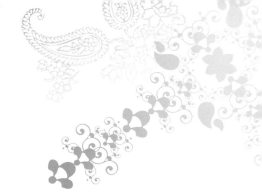

# Seated forward bend

– PASCHIMATTANASANA
Strengthens your entire spine, and stretches the back of your thighs, calves, hips, and lower back. Good for digestion and strengthens the liver and heart.

1.  Sit with hips parallel and legs extended. Grasp your big toes with your index fingers and thumbs. If you cannot reach with your legs straight, bend your knees slightly and squeeze your thighs so that you can keep your back as straight as possible. Breathe in, raise your chest, and draw your shoulder blades into the body. Sit steady, and press the pads of your feet slightly forward in order to engage the legs.

2.  Breathe out, and let your upper body fall forward over your legs. Keep your chest open, and broaden your shoulders so that you do not tense your shoulders or neck too much. Hold this position for five deep breaths. Feel the support from your deep abdominals, and raise your chest forward in the direction of your toes with the help of each exhalation.

3.  Breathe in, rise up with your chest keeping hold of your toes, and breathe out.

4.  Do a *Vinyasa*, and return to seated position. See the next page.

Between each side of the movement, or between each movement itself, you do a *Vinyasa*, or transition.

# Vinyasa

1.  Cross your feet, breathe in, and press against the floor, keeping all of your weight on your hands as you step or jump a leg's length back.

2.  Breathe out, and come down to the *Plank*. You may keep your knees on the floor if you need to.

3.  Breathe in, roll over on your toes, and rise up to the *Upward-facing dog*.

4.  Breathe out, roll over on your toes, and raise your hips. Place your feet on the floor, and rise up to the *Downward-facing dog* with your hips up and back and your head facing downward.

5.  Breathe in, and step or jump forward to crossed legs.

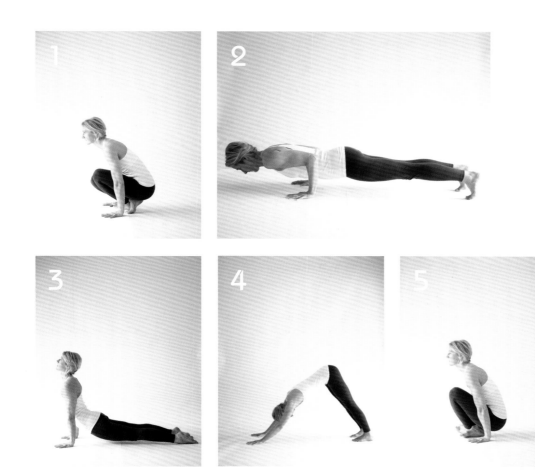

# Head to knee pose

– JANU SHIRSHASANA

Limbers up the ligaments in your feet, back, and ankles, and makes the joints in your knees and hips more flexible. Engages the spleen, liver, pancreas, and kidneys.

1. Sit in the starting position with legs extended. Move your right foot in toward the center of your body so that the knee is at a 90-degree angle to the hips. Grasp your left foot with both hands. Keep your knee bent if you need to. Breathe in, and stretch your chest upward.

2. Breathe out, and let your upper body fall downward and straight ahead from the hips. Then gradually come down toward your leg with your entire body, keeping one hand around the other in front of your foot. Keep your bottom on the floor, and let your breathing slowly extend your back forward. Hold this position for five deep breaths.

3. Breathe in, stretch your chest upward keeping hold of your left foot, and breathe out.

4. Do a *Vinyasa* (see page 36) and return to a seated position.

5. Now repeat the movement on the left side.

6. Do a *Vinyasa* (see page 36) and return to a seated position.

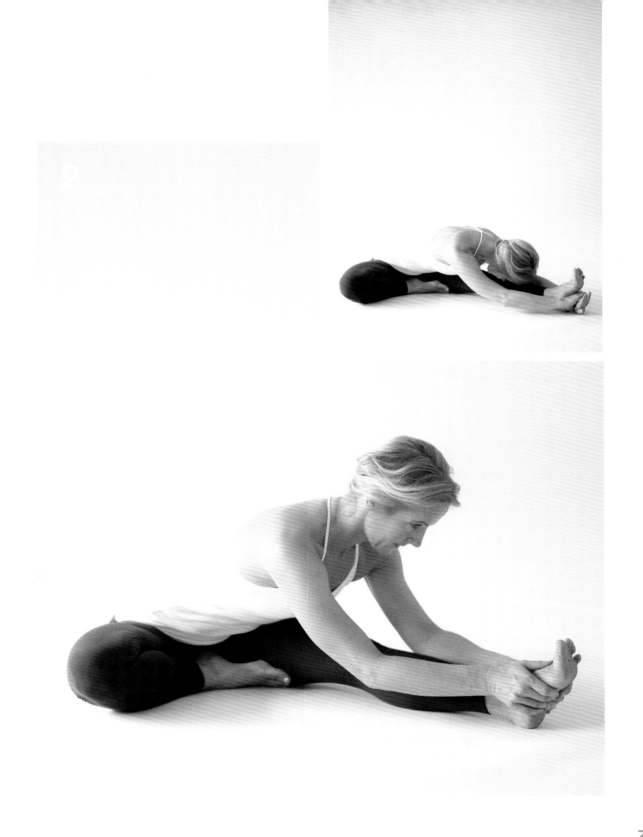

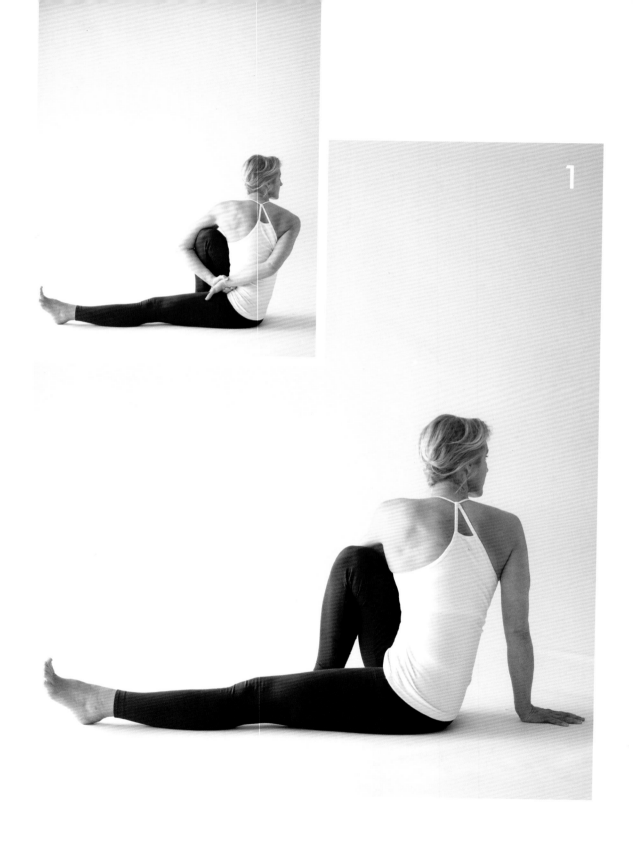

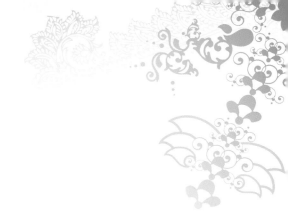

# Marichi's pose

– MARICHYASANA C

Relaxes the neural pathways in the spine, and increases mobility in the back. Makes the hips and shoulders more flexible. Cleanses and strengthens the kidneys, liver, spleen, and gall bladder. Beneficial for the intestines. Also strengthens the uterus.

1. Sit in the starting position with legs extended. Move your right foot in close to your bottom, with the foot at hips-width. Come over with your left elbow outside your right knee. Place your right hand behind your right hip, and look back over your right shoulder. Sit steady, and turn from your waist while raising and opening your chest. Hold this position for five deep breaths.

   As the movement grows, you can fix your left arm around your right leg, move your right arm behind your back, and grasp your hands together.

2. Breathe in, look forward again, hold your position, and breathe out.

3. Do a *Vinyasa* (see page 36) and return to a seated position.

4. Now repeat the movement on the left side.

5. Do a *Vinyasa* (see page 36) and return to a seated position.

# Boat pose

– NAVASANA
Strengthens your legs, hips, abdominal muscles, and lower back. Good for digestion.

1.  Sit in the starting position with legs extended. Lean back slightly, lift your legs, and raise your knees toward your upper body. Keep your arms extended straight ahead at shoulders-width apart. Open and stretch your chest forward. Be strong in your legs. Hold this position for five deep breaths. This position is called the *Boat*.

    As you become stronger, stretch out so that your legs are straight, but not at the expense of falling back and losing the strong center of your body.

2.  Place your hands on the floor beside your hips. Cross your feet. Breathe in, and press strongly with your hands against the floor so that you lift your body up off the floor. Breathe out, and come down again.

3.  Repeat the *Boat* three times, holding for five breaths each time. Do the small lift between each repetition.

4.  Do a *Vinyasa* (see page 36) and return to a seated position.

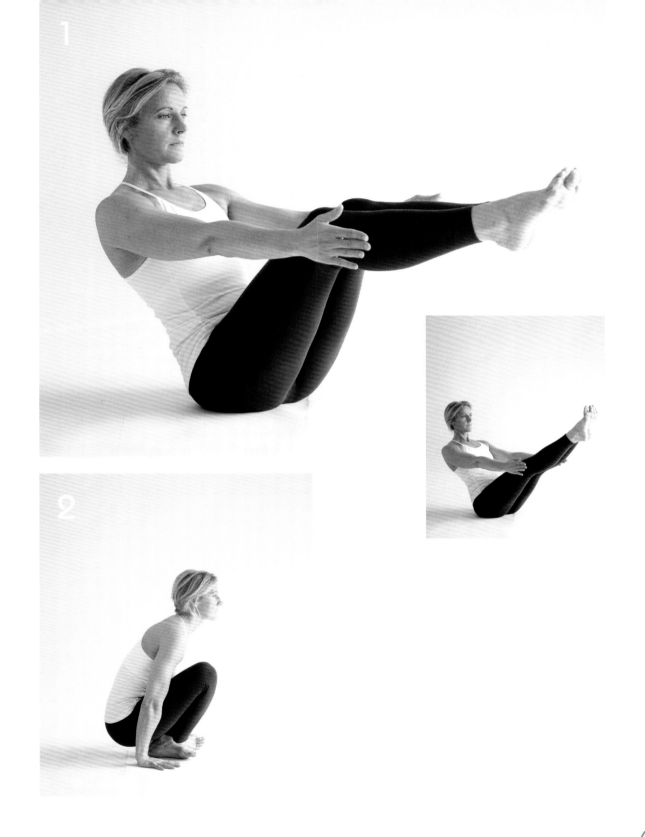

# Bound angle pose

– BADDHA KONASANA

Increases blood circulation and strengthens the entire lower abdomen. Opens up the hips and knees. Keeps the kidneys and bladder healthy. Prevents sciatica.

1. Sit in the starting position with legs extended. Breathe in, and move both feet as close to the center of your body as possible. Place your heels and soles together. Grasp your feet, and stretch your back upward so that you open your chest.

2. Breathe out, and let your upper body fall slowly toward the floor. Keep your bottom on the floor, feel support from your deep abdominals, and begin to lean your chest forward. Strive to come down with your chest toward the floor. Hold the position for ten deep breaths.

   If your knees point up toward the ceiling in this position, you may need to sit on a blanket or something similar. It also helps to have a wall behind you. In the beginning it will suffice to simply sit in this position and work on getting your knees down toward the floor. You can benefit from remaining in this position for a long time.

3. Breathe in, and rise up.

4. Do a *Vinyasa* (see page 36) and return to a seated position.

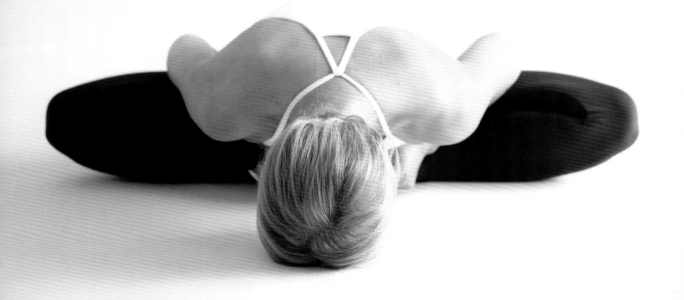

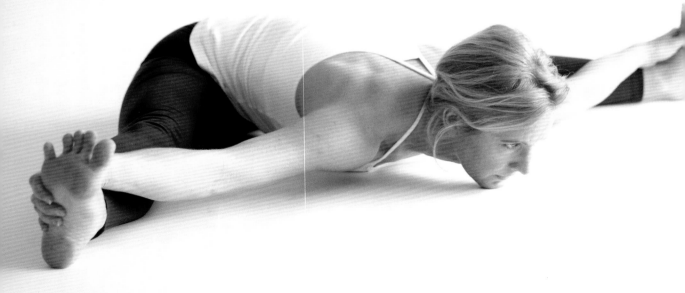

# Seated angle pose

– UPAVISHTHA KONASANA

Stretches the back of the thighs and hips. Opens the chest. Increases blood circulation in the entire lower abdomen, and keeps it healthy.

1.  Sit in the starting position with legs extended. Breathe in, and place your legs wide apart. Grasp the outsides of your feet, and raise your chest. Bend your knees if you cannot reach with your legs straight.

2.  Breathe out, and let your upper body fall toward the floor. Stabilize your bottom completely downward, and begin to lean your chest forward from the waist. Strive to come down with your chest toward the floor. Hold the position for ten deep breaths.

    If it seems difficult to let your upper body fall forward, you can place your hands behind your hips, and try to stretch your upper body upward so that your back is as straight as possible.

3.  Breathe in, and rise up.

4.  Do a *Vinyasa* (see page 36) and come down from the *Downward-facing dog* to lie on your stomach.

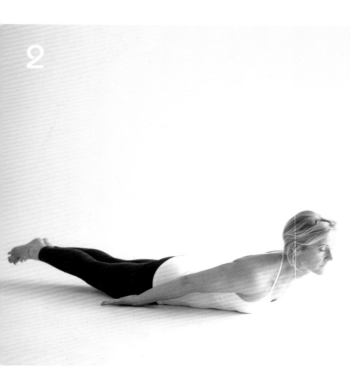

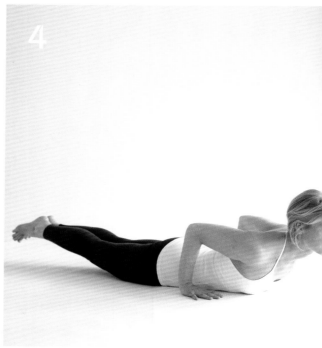

# Locust pose

– SALABHASANA

Helps digestion and counteracts flatulence. Makes the spine more flexible, and strengthens the lumbar region. Prevents the occurrence of a herniated disc.

1. Lie on your stomach, and keep your eyes on the floor with arms back along your sides and the backs of your hands on the floor.

2. Breathe in, and lift your head, chest, and legs up off the floor. Feel the strong support from your deep pelvic and abdominal muscles. Press your feet backward. Be strong in your legs, and keep your feet and knees together. Hold the position for five deep breaths.

3. Breathe out, come down again, and place your hands at waist-height with your palms on the floor.

4. Breathe in, and repeat the movement, now with your palms on the floor.

5. Do a *Vinyasa* (see page 36) and come forward from the *Downward-facing dog* to stand on your knees.

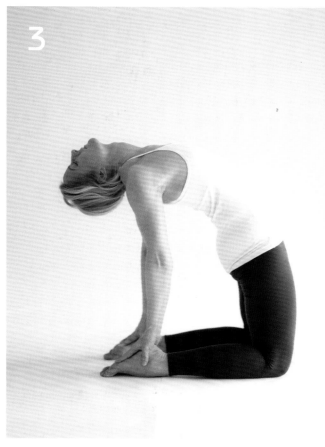

# Camel pose

– USTHRASANA

Opens the shoulders and chest. Strengthens and stretches your back and legs.

1.  Stand on your knees with knees at hip's width. Make sure that your feet are placed straight behind your knees. Try to spread your toes and feel both your big toes and your little toes on the floor. Be strong in your legs.

2.  Breathe in, place your hands on your hips, and push your hips forward. Keep contact with your deep pelvic and abdominal muscles. Roll your shoulders forward, broaden them, and raise your chest up high.

3.  Breathe out, move your hands back, and grasp your heels. Weigh down on them with your hands, and raise your chest high. Stretch your neck backward. Push your hips forward so that your back bends backward into an arch. Hold the position for ten deep breaths.

    If it is difficult to reach your heels, stay with your hands on your waist, bend your back backward as much as you can, and breathe there instead.

4.  Breathe in, and rise up again.

5.  Do a *Vinyasa* (see page 36) and return to a seated position.

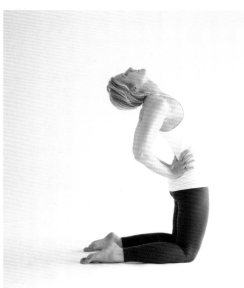

# Bridge pose

– SETU BHANDA SARVANGASANA
Strengthens your back, hips, and buttocks. Also strengthens your entire core around your pelvis, giving greater stability to the lumbar region and lower back, which are often weak areas in the back.

1.  Lie on your back, bend your knees, and place your feet hip-width apart directly below your knees. Your lower legs should be at 90-degree angles to your feet and knees. Your toes should point straight ahead, and your hips, knees, and toes should be in line. Push your lumber region down toward the floor so that your lower back is straight.

2.  Breathe in, and raise your pelvis, hips, and chest toward the ceiling. Roll your shoulders in slightly, and fold your hands on the floor below you. Press your arms down carefully so that you can lift your chest higher. Feel your big toes on the floor so that you have contact with the inside of your thighs, and in order to keep your knees from falling out to the side. Imagine your tailbone going forward between your knees so that you reduce the stress on your lumber region, and try to relax your buttocks. Hold the position for five deep breaths.

3.  Breathe out, come down, and rest for five breaths.

4.  Repeat the movement three times.

5.  Bend your knees toward your chest, squeeze your knees, and roll slowly from side to side in order to stretch your lumbar region.

6.  Come over on your side, and weigh down with your hand so that you rise up carefully to seated position.

    As you become more flexible and stronger in your back, you can try to rise up to the *Wheel*, which is described on the next page.

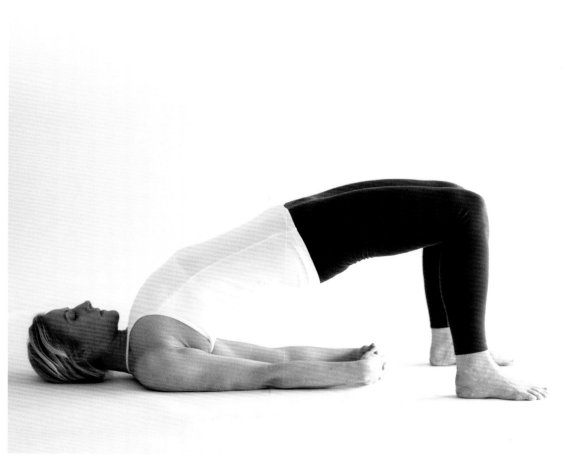

# Wheel pose

– URDHVA DHANURASANA

Strengthens, limbers up, and gives life to the spine. Also strengthens the arms and wrists. Gives greater life force and energy.

The *Wheel* is done in the same way as the *Bridge*, but for this pose you place your hands beside your ears and lift your body up from the floor so that only your hands and feet have contact with the floor. In the *Wheel*, you try to keep your arms as straight as possible so that your elbows do not fall out to the side. Let go of your neck entirely so that your head hangs freely.

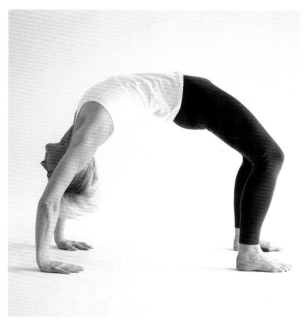

# Diagonal stretch

Releases tension in your back and neck. Opens your thorax and stretches your chest muscles.

1.  Lie on your back with knees bent, breathe out, and let your knees fall to the left. Keep your shoulder blades on the floor, and lay your arms over your body to the right. Rest your gaze over your arms, and hold the position for ten deep breaths.

2.  Breathe out, and now repeat the movement on the other side.

3.  Come over on your side, and push yourself up to a seated position with the help of your arm.

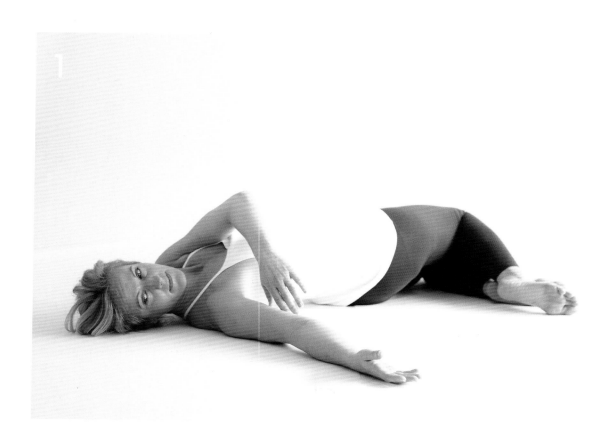

# Seated forward bend

– PASCHIMATTANASANA

Stretches the back of your thighs, calves, hips, and lower back, and refreshes the entire spine. Facilitates digestion, and strengthens the liver and heart.

1.  Sit with hips parallel, and extend your legs. Grasp the outsides of your feet with your hands. If you cannot reach with your legs straight, then bend them slightly. Breathe in, raise your chest, and draw your shoulder blades into the body. Stabilize your bottom on the floor and press the pads of your feet slightly forward so that you engage your entire legs.

2.  Breathe out, and let your upper body fall forward over your legs. Keep your chest open and broaden your shoulders so that you do not tense your shoulders or neck too much. Hold the position for ten deep breaths. Feel the support from your deep abdominals, and raise your heart forward in the direction of your toes with the help of each exhalation.

3.  Breathe in, rise up with your chest keeping your hands on your feet, and breathe out. Let go of your feet.

4.  Do a *Vinyasa* (see page 36) and return to a seated position.

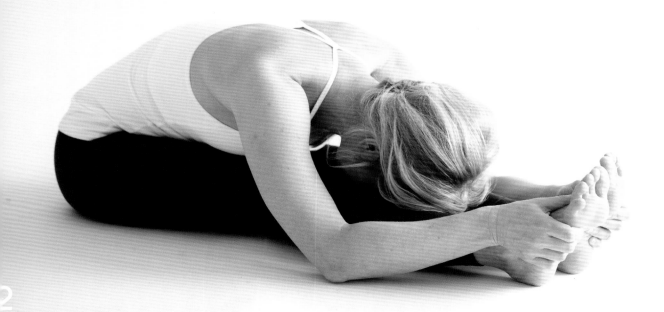

# Legs up the wall pose

before you can do the *Shoulder stand*

– VIPARITA KARNI
Relieves pressure on the back and counteracts tired and swollen legs.

1. Sit down beside a wall.

2. Roll down on your back while moving your legs up the wall. Make sure that your bottom is close to the wall, and keep your upper body straight. If you need to, place a pillow under your bottom for support. Extend your neck, and keep your chin slightly toward your chest. Relax your shoulders and neck.

3. Place your legs straight up, take ten breaths, then separate your legs outward and take an additional ten breaths. Finally, put the soles of your feet together, and take ten breaths.

4. Breathe out, and lower your legs from the wall. Come upright again on the mat, and go directly into the *Fish* pose (see page 56). Before you do the complete *Shoulder stand*, you must have built up adequate strength in the center of your body so that you are able to lift your legs up in the air with the help of the strength of your core. It is very important that you do not lie and weigh down on the cervical region of your spine. You must also be flexible in your neck and shoulders.

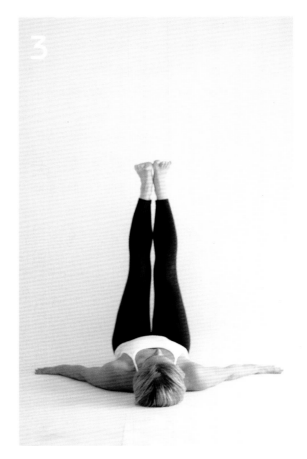

# Shoulder stand

– SALAMBA SARVANGASANA

One of yoga's main poses, *Shoulder stand* is said to cure all illnesses. The increased blood circulation is beneficial for all organs and hormones. The pose gives harmony and pleasure to the entire human system, and it is said to strengthen all the senses. It is also very helpful for breathing difficulties.

1. Lie flat and feel that you have contact with the base of your pelvis and your deep abdominals. Take a couple of breaths.

2. Breathe in, roll up onto your shoulders, and place your hands on your back for support.

3. Move your elbows in at shoulder-width apart, and lift your legs straight up toward the ceiling. You must rest on your shoulders and elbows. The back of your head also supports you against the floor, but the cervical region of your spine must be entirely free from weight against the floor. Feel the support from your inner abdominal lock, which lifts your legs upward. Hold the position for ten to twenty deep breaths.

4. Breathe out and roll down carefully using your arms for support against the ground. Then remain lying here in order to go directly into the next pose, the *Fish*, which is a countermovement to the *Shoulder stand*.

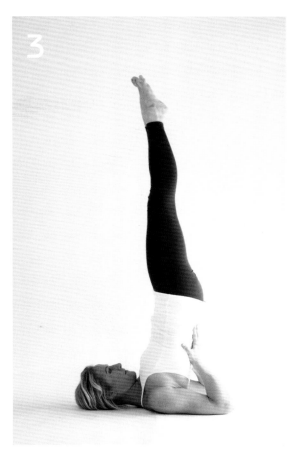

# fish pose

– MATSYASANA

This is a countermovement to the *Legs up the wall* pose and the *Shoulder stand*.
It makes the neck stronger and more flexible, opens the chest, and is good for the
heart and lungs.

1.  Lie down flat on the mat.

2.  Grasp the sides of your buttocks, and raise your chest toward the ceiling. Either
    stop here with your elbows on the floor and your neck stretched back, or fold
    the top of your head toward the floor. Hold this position for ten deep breaths.

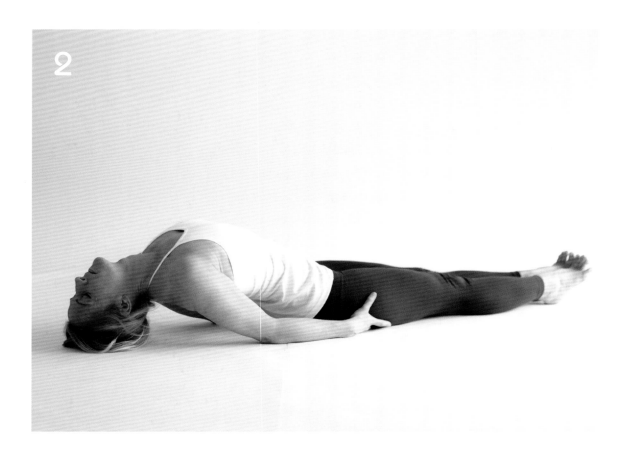

# Child's pose

– BALASANA
A very effective and deeply relaxing recovery pose that straightens out the back.

1.  Kneel down, and let your upper body fall forward over your knees. Rest your forehead on the floor, and keep your arms either in front of you with your palms on the floor or back along your sides. Try to come down with your buttocks toward the back of your thighs. Breathe deeply here for a while.

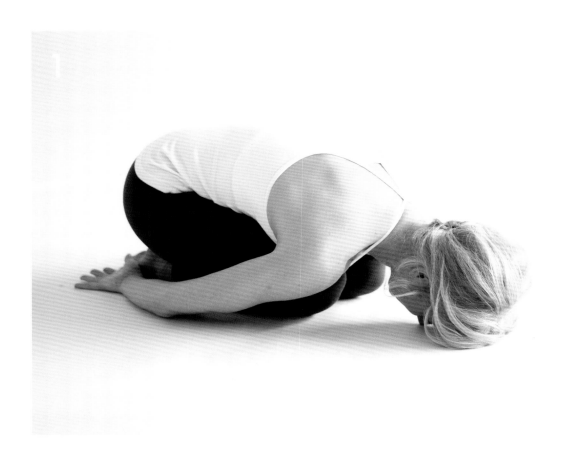

# Seated breathing, lotus pose

– PADMASANA

The king of the yoga poses and a perfect pose for meditation. It opens the hips, chest, and knees, and strengthens the back.

1. Sit down with legs crossed. If you have difficulty stretching your back upward, you can place a pillow or blanket under your bottom.

   You will eventually be able to sit in the *Lotus* pose. Lift your right foot up first, and then your left.

2. Feel support from your inner abdominals, and stretch your back upward. Keep your shoulders in line with your hips so that you do not lean forward or backward. Lower your chin slightly toward your chest, but keep the back of your neck extended.

3. Extend your arms, rest the backs of your hands on your knees, and keep your index fingers and thumbs together. Close your eyes, or rest your gaze on the tip of your nose. Hold this position for twenty-five deep breaths.

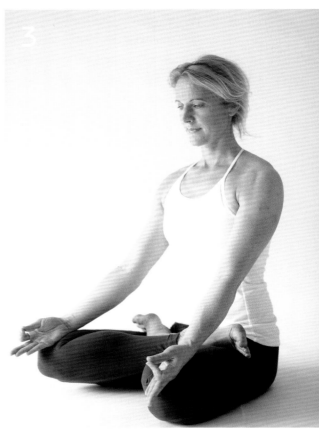

# Corpse pose

– SAVASANA

You must always make sure to have at least five minutes of total rest after a full yoga session. It is in rest that the body can incorporate the energy you have built up during the session.

Lie down flat on your back. Put a blanket over yourself, and close your eyes. Extend your legs, and let your feet fall to the side. Your arms should rest alongside your body, and your palms should open toward the ceiling. Lower your shoulders, and stabilize your body against the floor. Feel how your entire body slowly relaxes and rest in your body's weight. If a thought arises, let it merely pass, and listen instead to your breathing as it becomes calmer and calmer. Simply rest peacefully, and relax completely for a while.

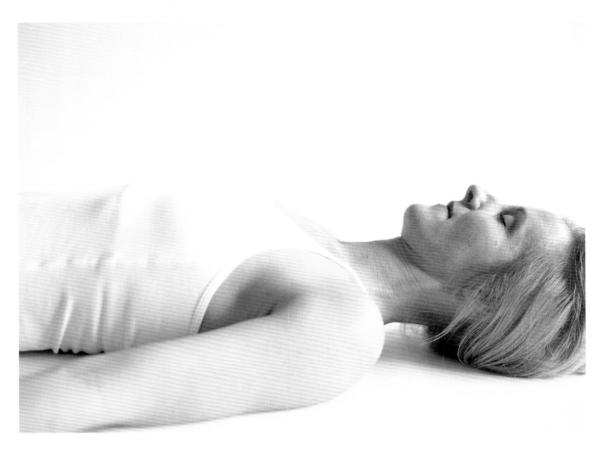

# Your yoga

Yoga is your friend in life. Take the time to embrace yoga fully and wholeheartedly and your body will slowly become stronger and more flexible, and your mind more at ease. Yoga is a path toward a more harmonious existence. With a strong body and a peaceful soul, it is easier to manage the everyday world with all its needs. Even situations that may otherwise seem difficult become easier to handle. Yoga helps you to focus on that which is important to you, and you will see that you become both kinder toward yourself and more humble in your surroundings.

For me, yoga is my own time: In yoga I can collect my thoughts and clear away those that are unnecessary. I always take some time before and after my yoga session to meditate over whatever feels important in life. I send my thoughts out to those in need and meditate over what I wish to take place. Try to take some time for yourself to sense how you feel today, and focus on what you wish and think. It's preferable to do that in connection with your yoga time, before or after you have sat breathing. If you do not have time to do your yoga sequence, then still try to take time each day to be in quietude, and to simply be together with yourself for a while.

Following tradition, in yoga we say a mantra before the session. The mantra honors and reveres the teachers who have led the yoga tradition and made it possible for us to do yoga today. In the mantra we will also discover our true selves by awakening the light that is found in us all. After yoga, we share among us the energy we have gained, and we send it out to all living things. It is a beautiful thought that I hope you can come to share and feel in your path through yoga.

# Opening mantra
Sanskrit

Oṃ!
vande gurūṇāṃ caraṇāravinde
sand arśita-svātmā-sukhāvabodhe
niḥśeyase jāṅgali-kāyamāne
saṃsāra-hālāhala-moha-śāntyai
ābāhu-puruṣāk āraṃ
śaṅkha-cakrāsi-dhāriṇam
sahasra-śirasaṃ śvetaṃ
praṇamāmi patañjalim
Oṃ!

OM
I bow before the lotus feet of the Gurus
who make clear the boundless happiness of
our soul.
The healer who removes the delusion,
the poison that is born of the cycle of life
and death.
The brightly shining Patanjali, with his head
of a thousand snakes
and the body of a man below the shoulders,
with a conch shell, a chakra, and
a sword in his hand, I respect deeply.

OM peace peace peace

# Closing mantra
Sanskrit

Oṃ!
svasti prajābhyaḥ paripālayantaṃ
nyāyena mārgeṇa mahīṃ mahīśāḥ
go-brāhmaṇebhyaḥ śubham astu nityaṃ
lokāḥ samastāḥ sukhino bhavantu

Oṃ śāntiḥ śāntiḥ śāntiḥ

OM
Let prosperity come,
let the soul and the body be nourished,
let the rulers reign justly over their land,
let peace and gentleness, knowledge and
godliness always prevail,
let happiness and goodness be found
throughout the world,
let the rain arrive in time and the earth give
ample harvest,
let fairness and freedom replace fear,
let the generations continue to be fertile and
let poverty come to an end,
let every man live one hundred healthy years.

OM peace peace peace

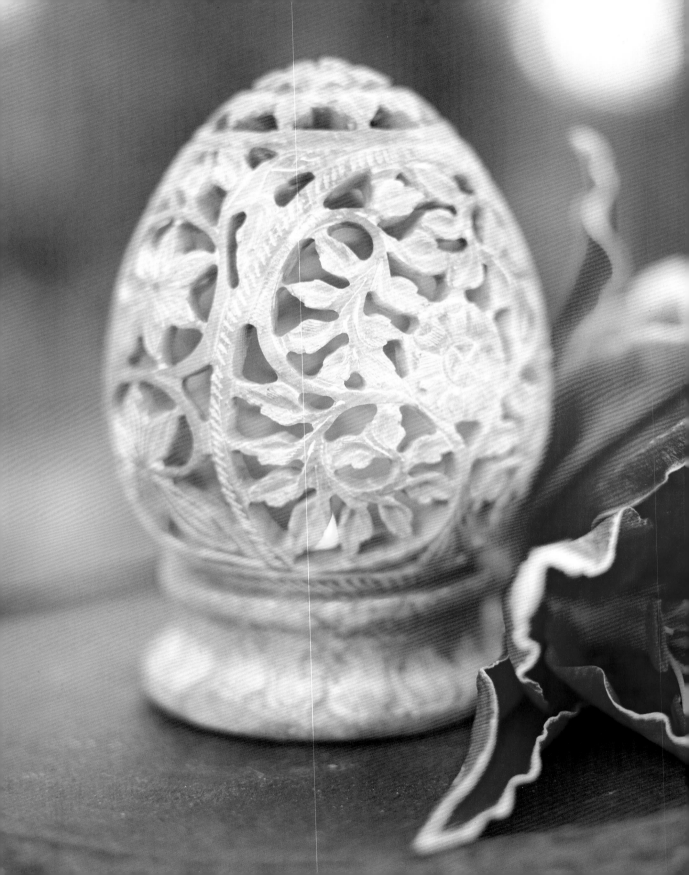

# Sun salutation A

# Sun salutation B

63

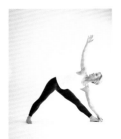

Utthita Trikonasana

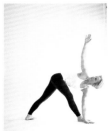

Parivritta Trikonasana

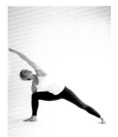

Utthita Parschrakonasana

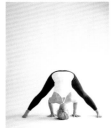

Prasarita Padottarasana A

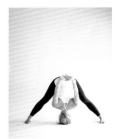

Prasarita Padottarasana B

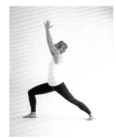

Virabhadrasana 1

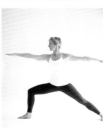

Virabhadrasana 2

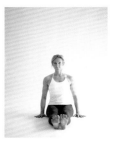

Dandasana

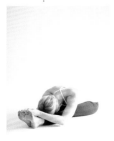

Paschimattasana

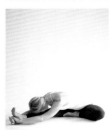

Janu Shirsasana

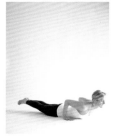

Marichyasana C

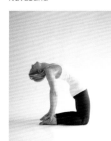

Navasana

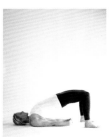

Baddha Konasana

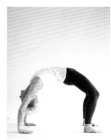

Upavishta Konasana

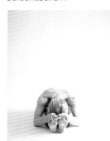

Salabhasana A

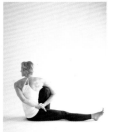

Salabhasana B

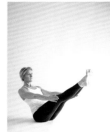

Usthrasana

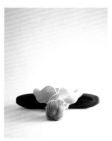

Setu Banda Sarvangasana

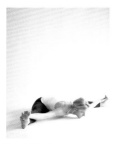

Urdhva Dhanurasana

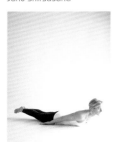

Paschimattasana

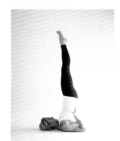

Salamba Sarvangasana

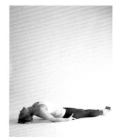

Matsyasana

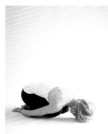

Balasana

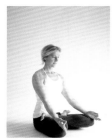

Padmasana

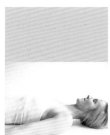

Savasana